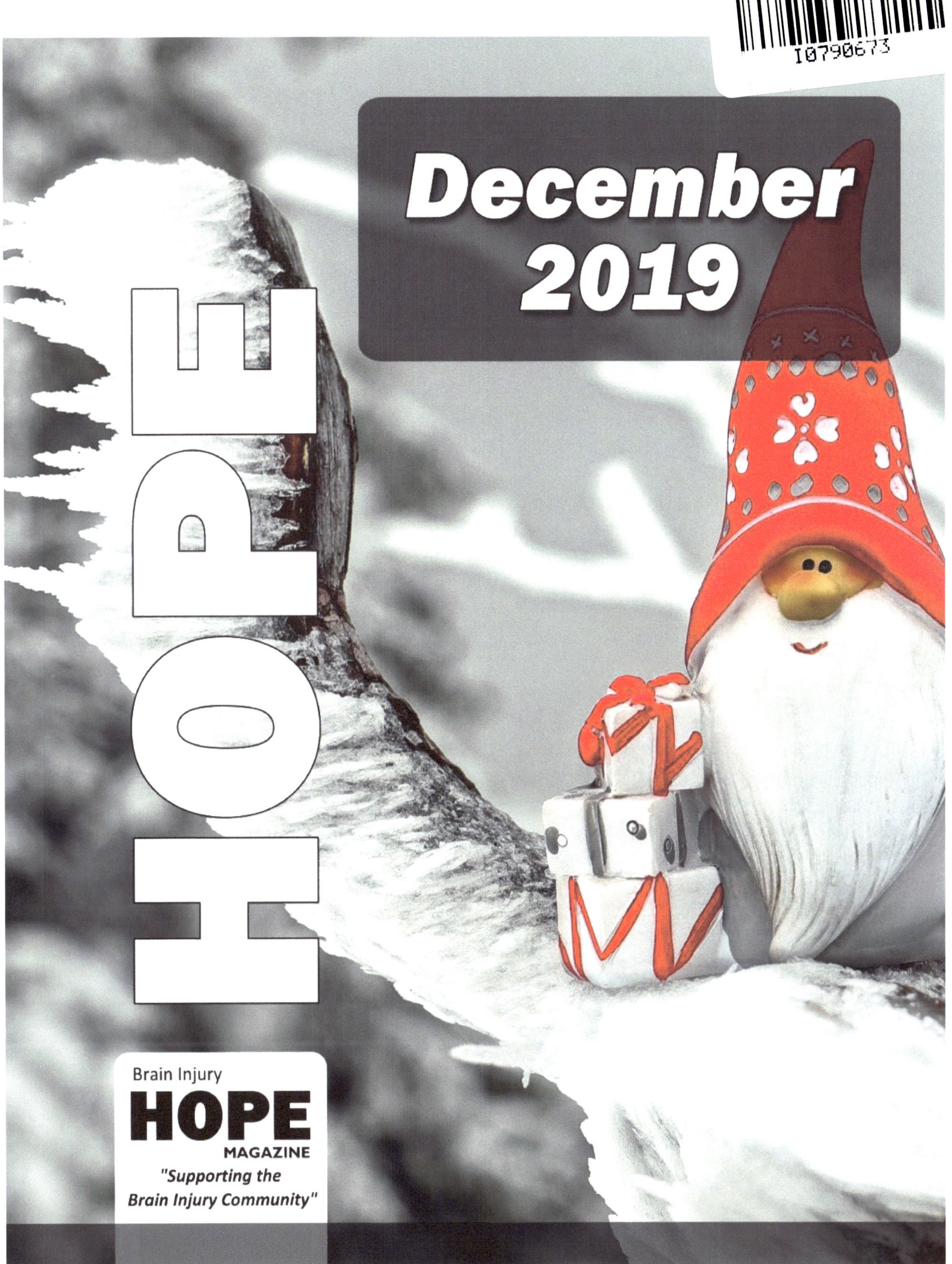
December
2019
HOPE
Brain Injury
HOPE
MAGAZINE
"Supporting the
Brain Injury Community"

Welcome

HOPE MAGAZINE

Serving the Brain Injury Community Since 2015

December 2019

Publisher
David A. Grant

Editor
Sarah Grant

Our Contributors

Patrick Brigham
Virginia Cote
Archie Fife
Deb Gorman
David A. Grant
Kelly Lang
Lisa Yee

Welcome to the December 2019 Issue of HOPE Magazine!

This month's issue of HOPE Magazine features a wonderful mix of new contributing writers as well as some of our perennial favorite contributors. Over the years, our readers have repeatedly said that they appreciate that the stories published in HOPE Magazine reflect the reality of life after brain injury *the way it really is.*

Realistically, no greater good is served by offering a candy-coated version of the reality of life after brain injury. It is all-to-often messy, difficult, and profoundly challenging. But life after everything changes can be full of unexpected victories, new friends, and a life that none of us ever expected to live. I can say this from immensely personal experience. In addition to publishing HOPE Magazine, I am also a brain injury survivor.

An important note about our publication as well. Starting in 2020, we are moving toward a larger, more content rich version of our magazine. Rather than publishing monthly, we will be publishing on a quarterly basis. Watch for new features coming in 2020. We are very excited about this change!

Happy Holidays,

David A. Grant
Publisher

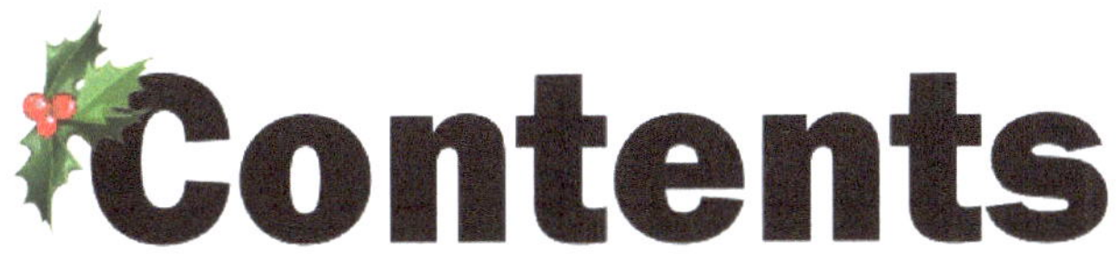

Contents

What's Inside This Issue

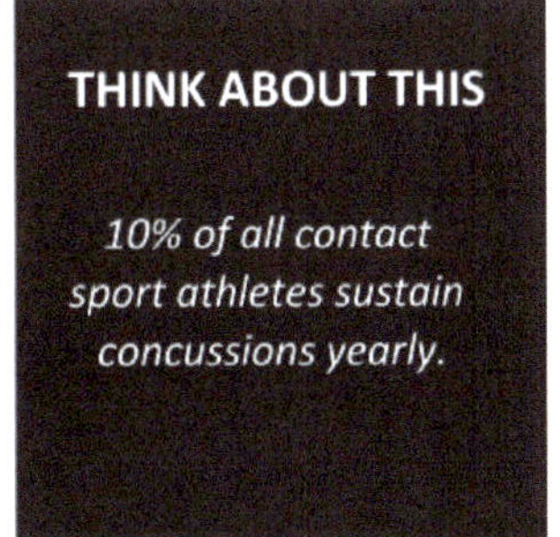

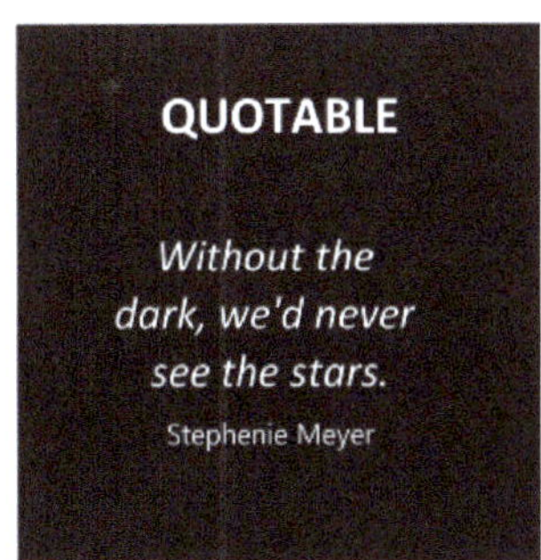

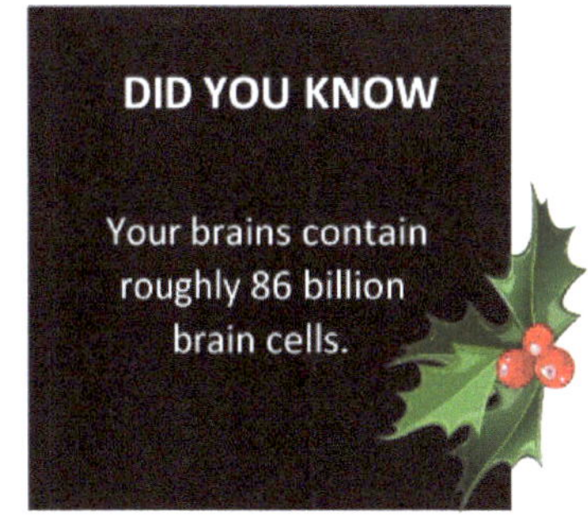

Story Callout: SUPPORT GROUPS

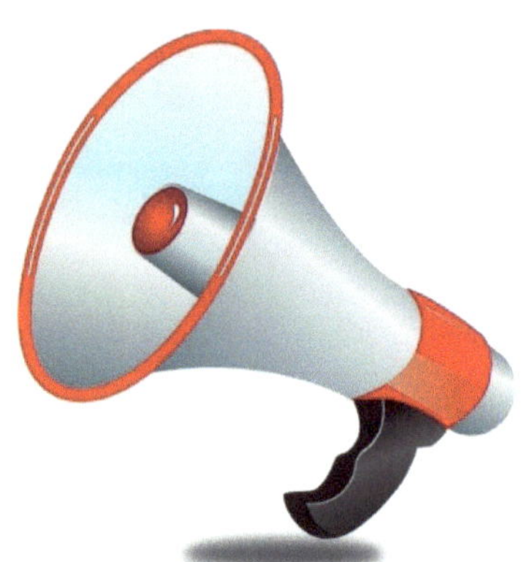

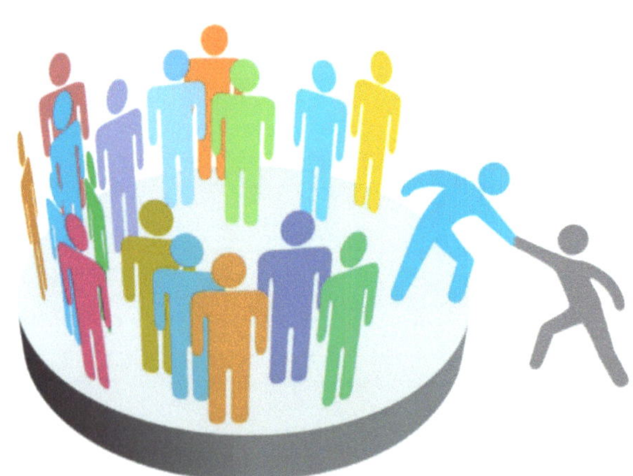

We are looking for stories for an upcoming issue of HOPE Magazine about your experience with Brain Injury Support Groups.

Support groups can and do save lives. An upcoming SPECIAL ISSUE of HOPE Magazine will be largely dedicated to this topic.

Your Story has Value!

And now the details...

- We prefer an article length of 800-1,000 words. Longer or shorter pieces will be considered.
- When submitting, please include a photo or photos to be included with your piece.
- Please include 2-3 photos to accompany your submission

Please email your submission to mystory@tbihopeandinspiration.com.

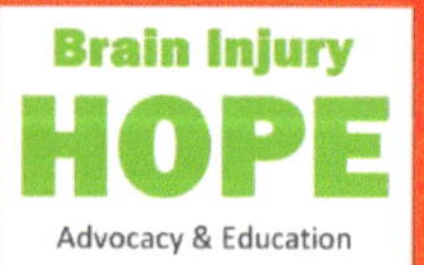

The Letter

By Debra Gorman

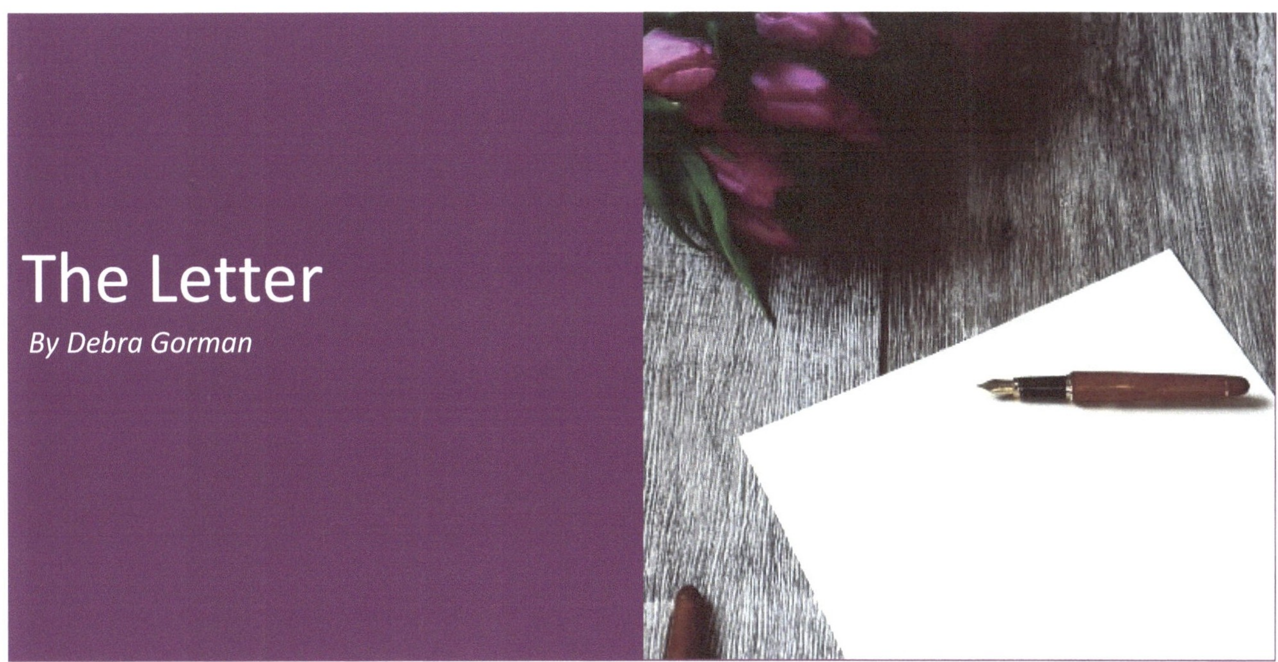

I recently listened to a podcast at 3:00 AM in the morning. I have hoped to be lulled back to sleep, but I was not. I heard something that I will find myself quoting for a long time. The guest on the podcast was recounting the story of a time she reluctantly confessed to a nosy stranger that she was battling cancer. The stranger offered her this advice: Don't hog your journey. It isn't just for you. What has happened is part of you. You can place your experience deep in your pockets or you can come alongside someone, sharing out of your knowledge and experience. It's your choice.

Isn't that profound? I realized that's exactly what I had been trying to do in my quest to extract meaning from my brain injury experience. The blog and the articles that I write are all attempts to come alongside others who are experiencing the thing all humans share – shared suffering and pain. It comes at differing times and in different forms, but pain is pain, whether it is physical, emotional or spiritual.

> *"You can place your experience deep in your pockets or you can come alongside someone, sharing out of your knowledge and experience."*

I say that, and believe it, but I have also failed to live it out consistently. I would like to share an excerpt from a letter I wrote to my husband while he was away on a business trip. I gave it to him when he returned home:

"It hit me today with substantial force that I have wronged you over the last year and three months. I hope you will forgive me.

When I first learned you were going to survive your bike accident and subsequent brain injury, I was so relieved for you, and for us. Then, almost immediately my thoughts turned to me. Finally, you will have a better understanding of what I go through, how I feel, my difficulties.

Just last night I found myself ignoring your complaints. Often, I have said to myself when you mention an ailment, you have no idea how bad it could be. You are one of the fortunate ones. I wish you would buck up and be tough—like me. It's true, I seldom complain—out loud. However, I am affected every moment that my eyes are open, and I know I don't always handle my struggles well.

I have been a big proponent of the belief that suffering of any type is pain, and pain is a great equalizer of people. Who am I to say that my pain is worse than yours, or anyone else's? That is what I say I believe, but my behavior has suggested otherwise. I have not shown you the empathy or concern you deserve.

I have never heard you even hint at it, but you could easily have said to yourself, having a brain injury sucks. Thankfully, I have someone at home who has been through this and will understand me. If you said that to yourself, I am sorry for letting you down. I have failed you.

I realize my error now and intend to make amends. I love you so much and am so grateful to still have you in my life. Thank you for the way you love me, encourage, affirm and support me. Because of you, I'm glad to still be alive. I'm very happy to celebrate fourteen years of our marriage next month, sixteen years as a couple. Half of that time I have been brain injured. If we can keep from further scrambling our brains, we may celebrate a few more anniversaries."

I think I'm doing better since I had this awakening. I still believe that to truly love and enjoy life, we must discover meaning and purpose in it. I know many people who are living their best life, using the gifts God has given them to be a blessing in this world. As long as we draw breath, we have opportunity and purpose.

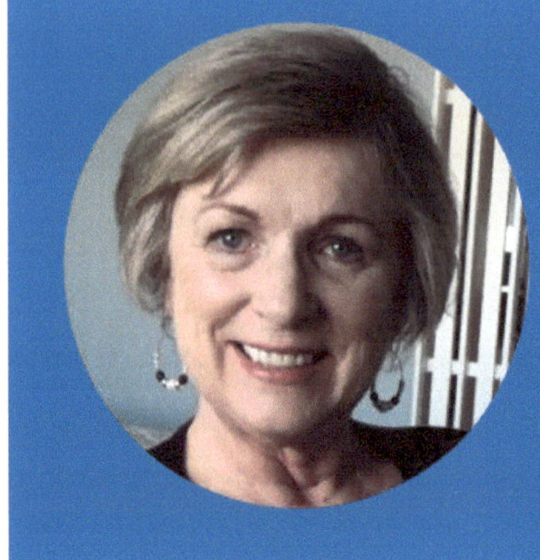

Meet Debra Gorman

Debra Gorman was fifty-six years old in 2011 when she experienced a cavernous angioma on her brain stem, causing her brain to bleed. Four months later she sustained a subdural hematoma. She later learned that she also had suffered a stroke during one of those events. She finds a creative outlet in writing. She enjoys writing for her children and grandchildren and has written articles that have been published for hospice, local newspapers, and Hope magazine. Currently, she writes for her blog, entitled Graceful Journey at debralynn48.wordpress.com.

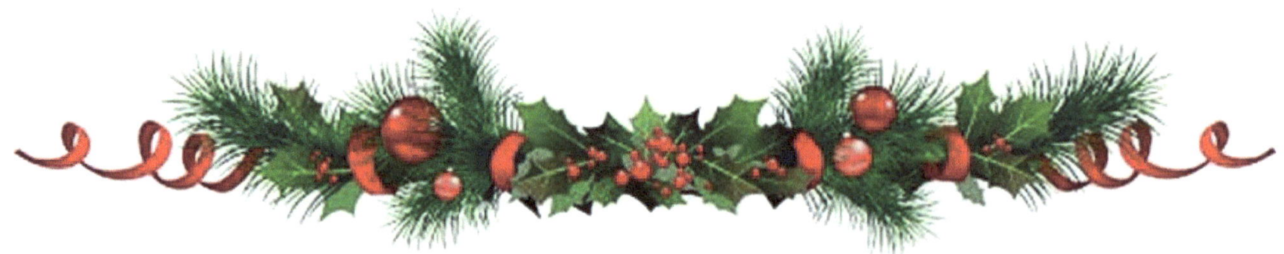

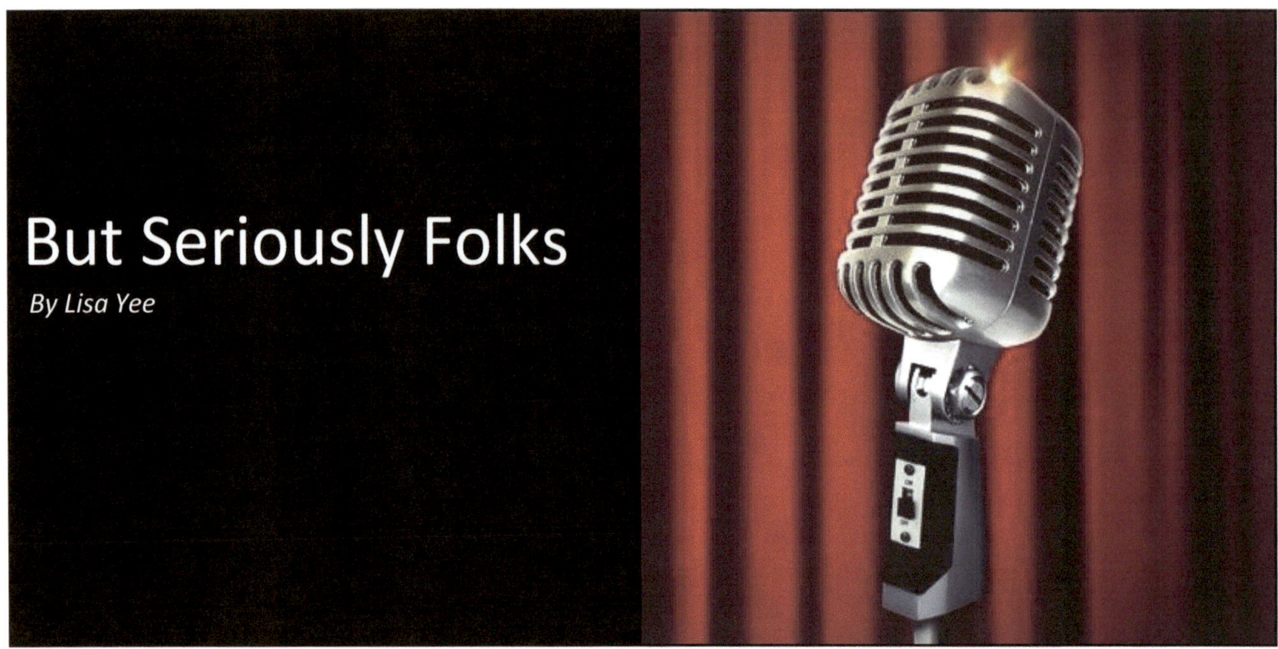

But Seriously Folks

By Lisa Yee

I have written quite a bit about what I call *the lighter side of brain injury,* but sometimes I worry that I'm giving TBI a good name. Living with brain trauma isn't as much fun as I may have been making it sound. As the politicians say, "Let me be clear." A lot of the time, it sucks. And I'm one of the lucky ones.

It's just that it's in my nature to play down the negative and see the humor in things. Thank God my sense of humor didn't get lost in the car crash with my recent memories, mathematical ability, and my directional sense.

So, what was I writing about? Oh, yes, the sucky side of brain injury. Well, dang it. So many TBI patients have it so much worse. I've seen the blogs. I've read the articles. My neurologist considers me a miracle. I am.

> *"Thank God my sense of humor didn't get lost in the car crash with my recent memories, mathematical ability, and my directional sense."*

Today I didn't wake up until almost 12:30 P.M. I felt like what I recall being hungover feels like. Yesterday I had allowed my senses to get overloaded. After yoga, a group of us met for lunch to celebrate a classmate who is finishing up rehab from a quadruple bypass he had in November. Our yoga class is like a big family, and we were all eager to welcome him back into the fold.

But the restaurant was actually a sports bar. Loud music, numerous screens showing sports events, and multiple conversations with multiple groups of friends proved to be too much. I had a good time, but to survive I took two breaks and intentionally zoned out for a while.

I was bummed out today after finally having my cereal, coffee and newspapers - plus social media, of course. By then it was midafternoon. Just then, I heard the little clicking sound on my phone that let me know that I had just received a text. It was my "little" brother. At forty-two, he's not so little anymore. "Just wanted to say hi. It occurred to me that I may not have told you I've been keeping up with your blog. Well, now I have."

Life is good. No joke.

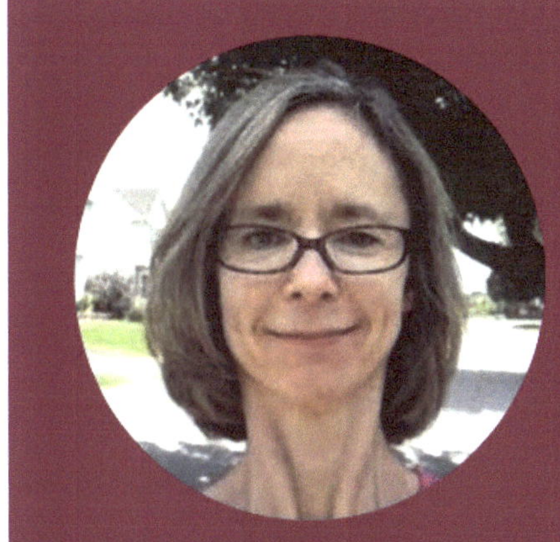

Meet Lisa Yee

Lisa, who lives in suburban Chicago, suffered a traumatic brain injury and acquired epilepsy in a 2008 car accident. For the previous two decades, she had worked in newspaper editing in Florida, North Carolina and Illinois. She and husband Ted have a daughter, Megan, of Chicago. Post-TBI, Lisa became certified as a yoga instructor and now volunteers teaching yoga at a women's shelter and a veteran's center.

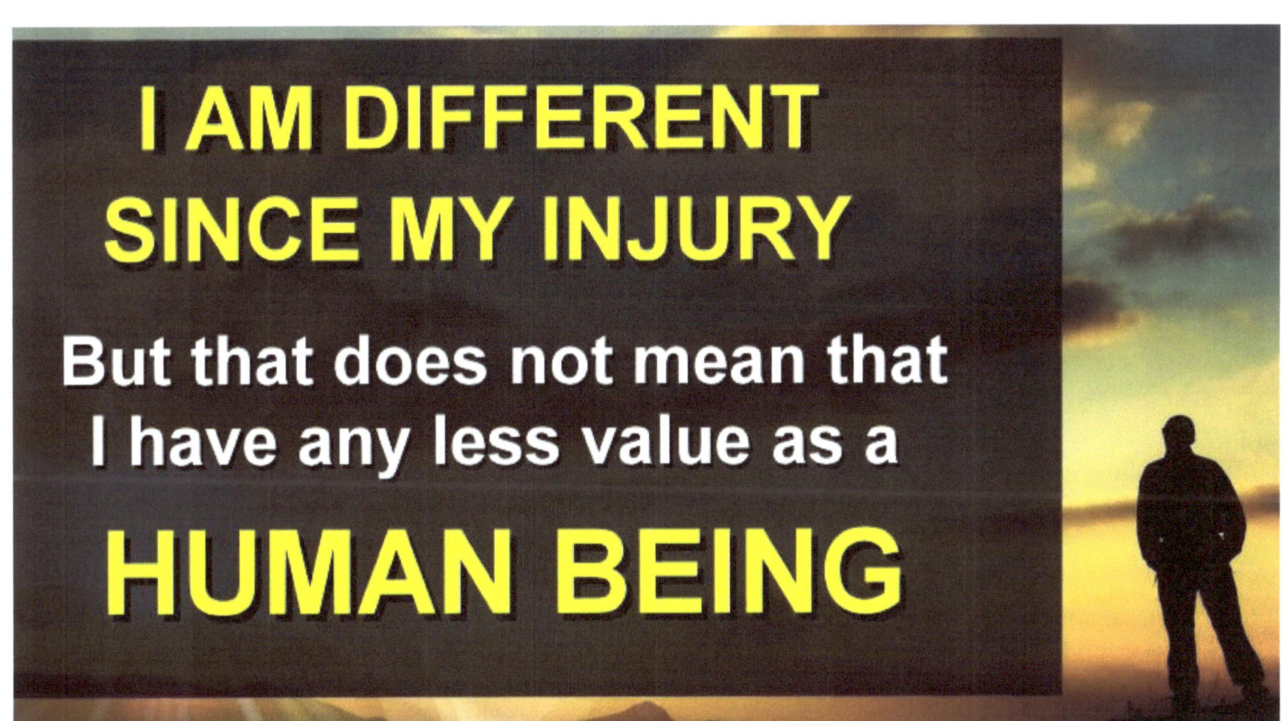

Help Wanted: Gategeeper

By Kelly Lang

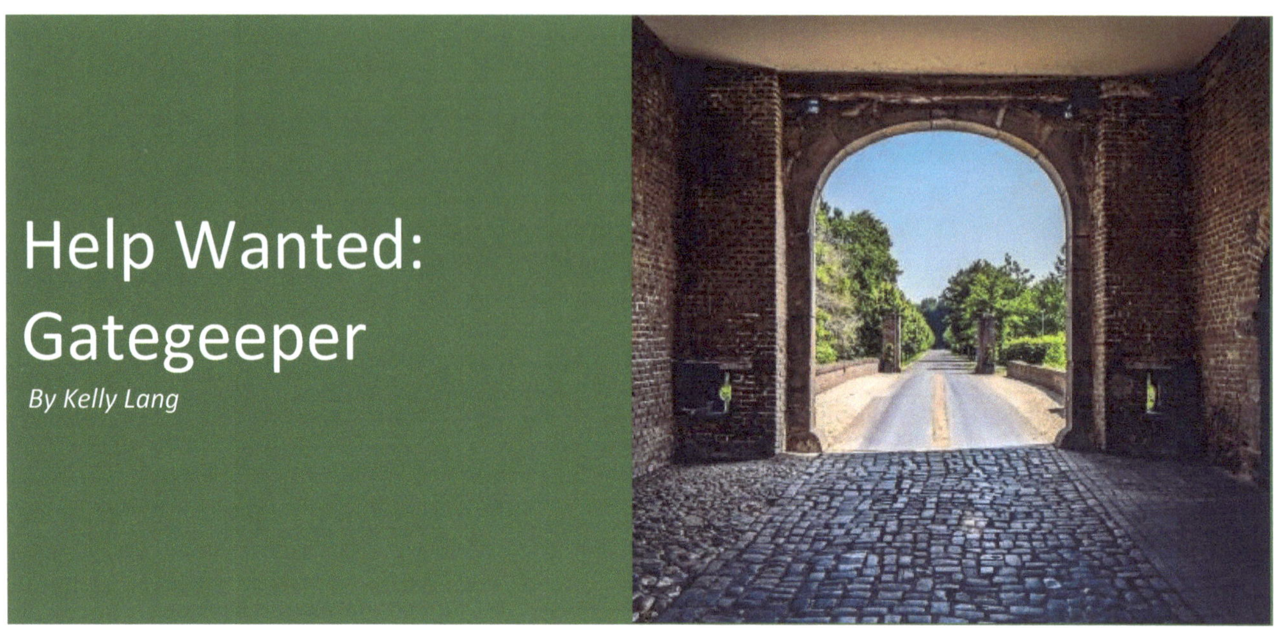

Discharge day was finally here. Even though the rehabilitation stay had only lasted two weeks instead of the six to nine months initially estimated, we were very anxious to leave. Departing the cold and sterile environment and returning to our life was all we wanted. Surprisingly it looked to be a beautiful day outside despite being the twenty-eighth of December in Baltimore. I kept Olivia entertained as much as possible between therapy sessions while we waited for discharge instructions.

Looking back, I compare this to what a prisoner must feel on their day of emancipation. While this may be a bit of an exaggerated metaphor, but many survivors and caregivers may relate.

How many of us have approached our "return to life" enthusiastically only to become despondent with all the things needed to do once we arrived home? Medical professionals explained the window of recovery was small and the more therapy a patient receives at the beginning stages of recovery, the more likely healing will occur. How were we going to coordinate all these efforts? There must be a leader who can direct us to all the services we need. Well, no there isn't.

> *"In many cases, ophthalmologists, orthopedists, dentists, and many more professionals have to be secured, insurance coverage verified, and most important, experience with brain injury investigated."*

We weren't told who to follow up with when we left the facility. We repeatedly asked the discharge doctor what needed to do once we settled in. After pressing him multiple times he finally relented and replied we should contact a pediatric neurologist as well as our primary care physician. Had we not pushed for this information we would have walked out not knowing where to turn.

It turns out we needed more than a primary care physician and neurologist. Therapists had to be found. In many cases, ophthalmologists, orthopedists, dentists, and many more professionals have to be secured, insurance coverage verified, and most important, experience with brain injury investigated. If the provider does not accept insurance or isn't covered under the plan other arrangements have to be made.

We carefully logged all of these appointments into our calendars so as not to forget where and when we need to be. Realizing how much work it takes to get our loved one in the car, packing supplies to feed and entertain while sitting in waiting rooms, navigating traffic was exhausting. I am exhausted just writing about the process.

I am brought back to the early days of my daughter's discharge. It was sobering once the euphoria of being home wore off and the realization of all the work awaiting us. It was not an easy task finding pediatric physical, speech and occupational therapists within a 20-mile radius who accepted our insurance, were knowledgeable about brain injury, and had openings in their schedules. Her name remained on many waitlists for months, and in some cases, even years.

The task was daunting, and I felt defeated more often than not. Looming over me were the words I heard in the hospital, "The first two years are the most vital in her recovery. Whatever progress she made had to occur during this timeframe." I was so consumed with worry as I pounded the phones. This was in 2002 and information was not readily available on the internet. I had to call individual offices and speak to receptionists, request recommendations from other doctor offices, and look in the phone directories.

I wasn't aware of any support groups for parents nor was I aware of any other resources to tap into. The inpatient rehabilitation was in a different state so I couldn't fall back on the facility for advice.

"I wasn't aware of any support groups for parents nor was I aware of any other resources to tap into."

Every doctor we visited wanted to know who else treated our daughter and what their impressions were or the treatment plan for her injury and subsequent issues. I felt like a broken record reciting the information over and over. I remember my husband, Mike, and I talking about finding a gatekeeper who could manage her care.

Someone we could call when a new issue arose, recommend providers, and communicate with all

> *According to dictionary.com a gatekeeper is a person in charge of a gate, usually to identify, count, supervise, etc., the traffic or flow through it. guardian; monitor.*

those involved in her treatment. We asked our brain injury case manager, doctor offices, parents at support groups but no one could give us an answer. Apparently, this individual did not exist. We tried getting all the providers under the same practice but that was futile as well.

Eighteen years later and we are still searching for the gatekeeper. Oh, I guess that person is me. I have managed to piece together a treatment team hoping they communicate with each other and when they do not, I provide the necessary information. It isn't always easy, but I do the best I can.

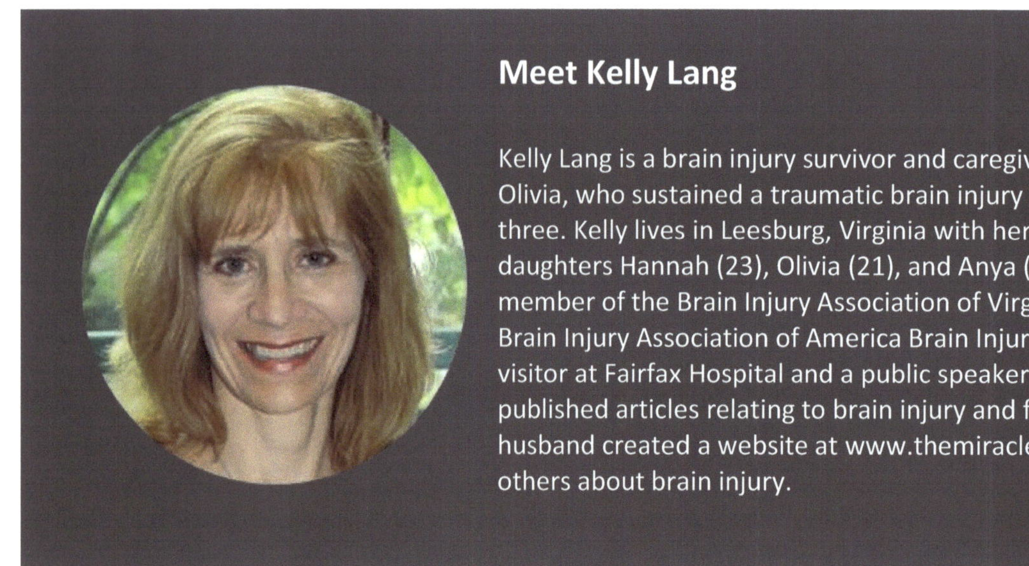

Meet Kelly Lang

Kelly Lang is a brain injury survivor and caregiver to her daughter, Olivia, who sustained a traumatic brain injury in 2001 at the age of three. Kelly lives in Leesburg, Virginia with her husband Michael, daughters Hannah (23), Olivia (21), and Anya (11). Kelly is a board member of the Brain Injury Association of Virginia, member of the Brain Injury Association of America Brain Injury Council, peer visitor at Fairfax Hospital and a public speaker. Kelly has also published articles relating to brain injury and family. Kelly and her husband created a website at www.themiraclechild.org to educate others about brain injury.

Love is the master key that opens the gates of happiness.

— Oliver Wendell Holmes Sr.

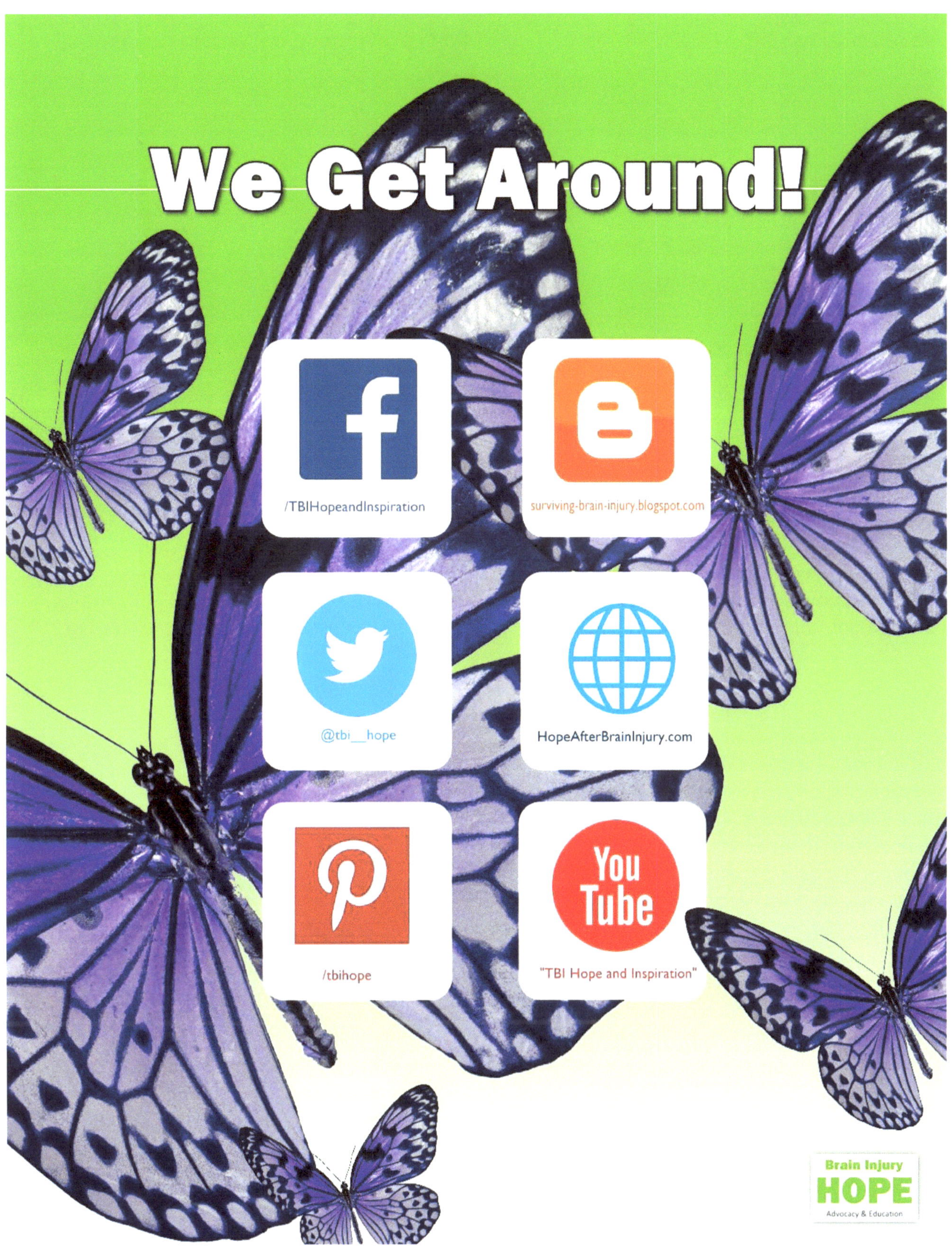

We Get Around!
/TBIHopeandInspiration
surviving-brain-injury.blogspot.com
@tbi__hope
HopeAfterBrainInjury.com
/tbihope
"TBI Hope and Inspiration"
Brain Injury
HOPE
Advocacy & Education

My New Life

By Archie Fife

I lived a fairly normal life growing up in Northeastern Pennsylvania with my dad, mom, sister and brother. I enjoyed spending time with my family. I was a laid back guy who enjoyed golf, fishing, playing pool, camping and spectator sports like car racing. I loved my job working seventeen to eighteen hours a day driving trucks.

Driving my big rig is how I was injured. I was driving my truck in white-out conditions when I hit the back of another truck. It took the emergency crew two hours to cut me out of my truck. I was airlifted to the hospital and was in the operating room for two days and in the hospital for a year. I spent nine months in a coma. I had to learn everything from the beginning. I had to learn to walk, eat and talk. My personality totally changed, and my anger was out of control.

> *"I was driving my truck in white-out conditions when I hit the back of another truck. It took the emergency crew two hours to cut me out of my truck."*

I would fight with everybody. It didn't matter who it was, why or what for. I even broke one nurse's fingers and another nurse's wrists and never realized I was doing it. My brain played tricks on me. For example, once I walked down the driveway to a highway and I was going to walk out in the middle of the highway thinking the traffic would just go right through me and wouldn't even bother me.

The staff that worked with me at the time had to catch me and stop me as I was walking towards the highway. Once the staff sat down and talked with me, I realized what I was about to do was wrong, but without their intervention I never would have seen that it was wrong. Brain injury does not just play tricks on your mind, it affects you in many ways. For me, my anger control, my short-term memory, my mood stability and judgement were my biggest issues. It took quite a while and hard work to learn how to deal with these issues.

It will not take days or weeks to fix my issues after brain injury, it took many years to figure out how to live my life satisfactorily and as close to normal as possible. ReMed, a brain injury rehabilitation and supported living system, helped save my life. If I didn't end up there, I would have been locked away in a mental institution. I have lived at ReMed for twenty-two years in various residential settings. I've even had the chance to get married with the support those who have helped with my care over the last two decades. This year, in October, celebrated my ten year wedding anniversary!

These days, I volunteer at a therapeutic horseback riding program. I walk with and lead horses so that people who have disabilities can have the freedom to ride horses. Living with a brain injury and the issues that come along with the injury is not easy. It is an invisible injury where people cannot see or tell which challenges you face. However, with hard work and patience you can still live a fairly normal life.

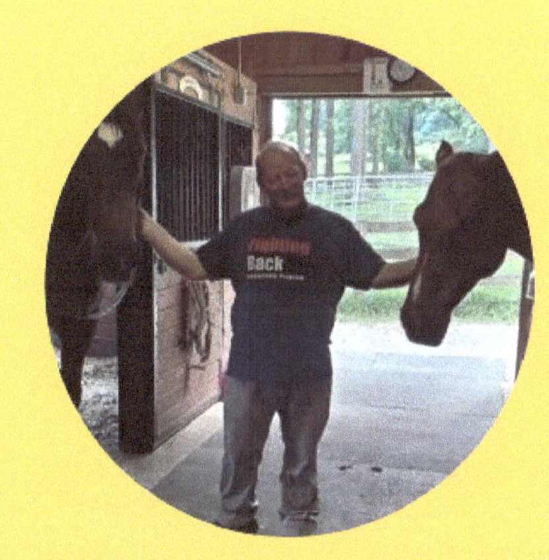

Meet Archie Fife

Archie Fife is a sixty-two year old man who lives in Malvern, PA. Archie lives at at a group home with other people who have traumatic brain injuries. He has been through lots in his life and has accomplished many things. He hopes to inspire others with his story.

"Renewal requires opening yourself up to new ways of thinking and feeling"

— Deborah Day

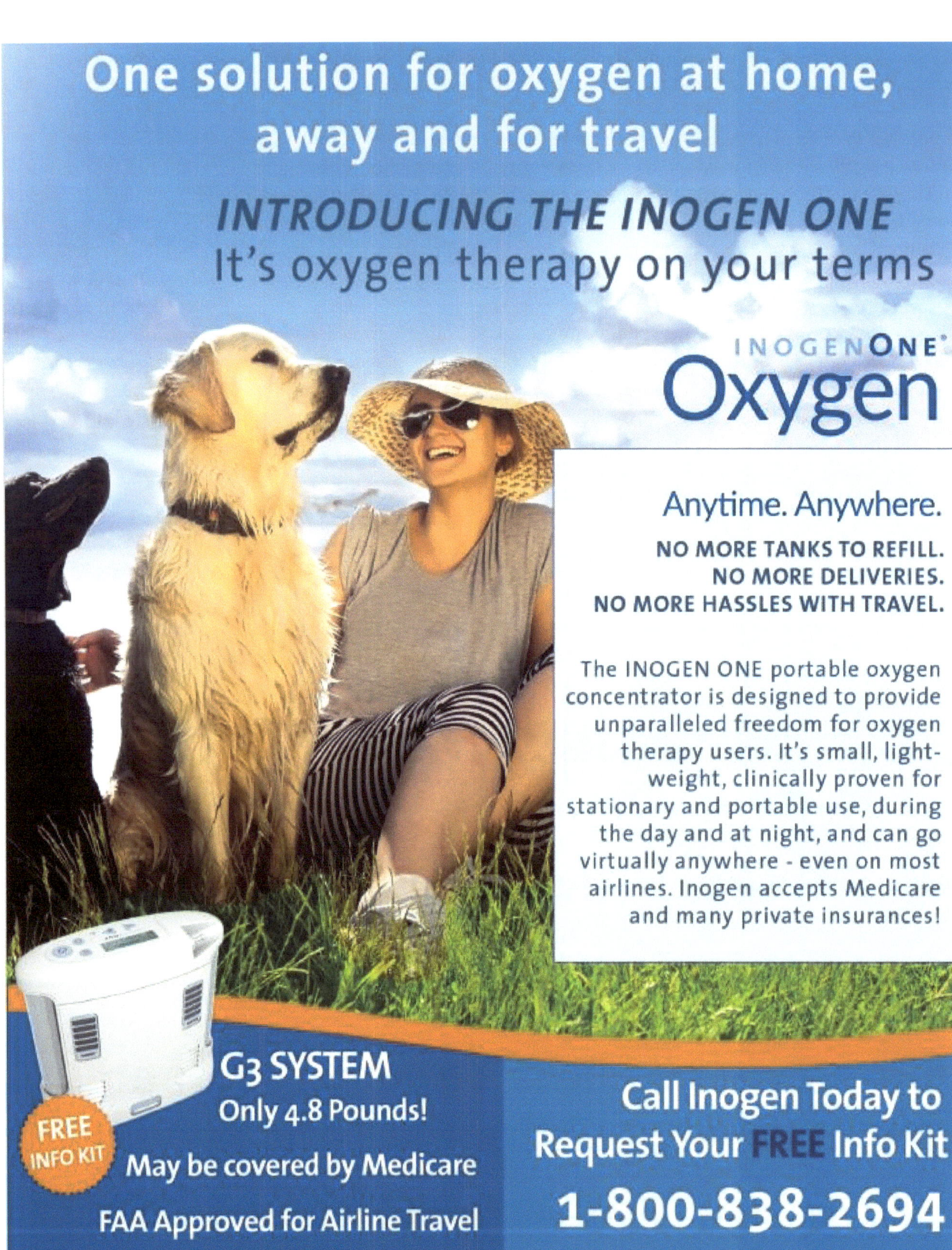

One solution for oxygen at home, away and for travel

INTRODUCING THE INOGEN ONE
It's oxygen therapy on your terms

INOGENONE®
Oxygen

Anytime. Anywhere.
NO MORE TANKS TO REFILL.
NO MORE DELIVERIES.
NO MORE HASSLES WITH TRAVEL.

The INOGEN ONE portable oxygen concentrator is designed to provide unparalleled freedom for oxygen therapy users. It's small, light-weight, clinically proven for stationary and portable use, during the day and at night, and can go virtually anywhere - even on most airlines. Inogen accepts Medicare and many private insurances!

G3 SYSTEM
Only 4.8 Pounds!
May be covered by Medicare
FAA Approved for Airline Travel

FREE INFO KIT

Lightweight Portable Oxygen Concentrator

Call Inogen Today to Request Your FREE Info Kit
1-800-838-2694

Reclaim your Freedom and Independence
MKT-P0035

A Family Affair

By David A. Grant

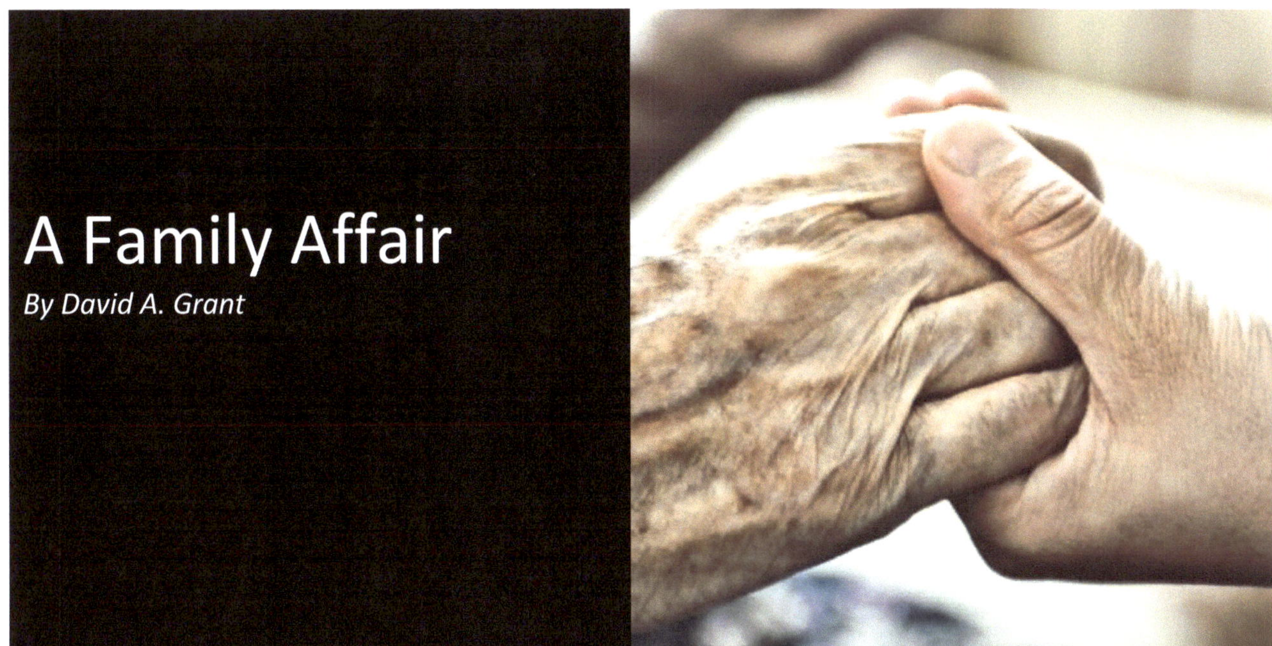

My mom passed away this past September. A little over two short months ago, the small church in her quiet New Hampshire town was filled to overflow capacity by those who knew and loved my mom. It was a touching tribute to a woman who touched the lives of so many.

In the early years after my own brain injury, in my innocent naivete, I thought that all brain injuries were traumatic brain injuries. It was only after several years of being part of the brain injury community that I learned otherwise. Acquired brain injuries are more commonplace than I ever knew. My Mom's final chapter started with an acquired brain injury.

Her stroke was a year ago, and thus began a year of institutionalization at a local rehab.

> *"Five years ago, I was not the person that I am today, as I wandered through my day-to-day life under the heavy cloak of brain fog."*

The last year has been one of the most bittersweet of my life. My wife Sarah and I were perhaps the most predominant caregivers for Mom. As a trip to her rehab was close to a 200-mile round trip, we secured a small lakeside rental for most of her last year. We were ever-present fixtures by her side. For the first time ever, I was able to see brain injury through a caregiver's perspective, offering me more insight as to what Sarah experienced after my injury.

"Thank goodness this was not five years ago," I said to Sarah countless times. Five years ago, I was not the person that I am today, as I wandered through my day-to-day life under the heavy cloak of brain fog. Mom's stroke and subsequent time at the rehab came at a time that I was able to actually be present, to be useful, and to help make critical decisions about her healthcare.

My own experience as a brain injury survivor gave me stunning insight into the challenges Mom faced. I was able to recognize slow processing and word-finding challenges for what they were – not because I was told by a healthcare provider, but because they were part of the very fabric of my own life. I find myself reflecting over a lifetime of memories.

When my first book, *Metamorphosis, Surviving Brain Injury*, was published, I was reluctant to let Mom read it. In an effort to spare my parents worry, I lied quite often during my first post-injury year. I did this to protect them. In my book, I was painfully candid about my struggles. My dad later told me that Mom spent several days crying after she completed reading my book. I was both devasted and relieved at the same time. Devasted in knowing that Mom anguished over my suffering, yet relieved that I no longer had to candy-coat how tough it really was.

Back in 2013, I presented in a keynote capacity at a Brain Injury Association of America annual conference in Maine. My mom and dad were in the front row. "David, we are so proud of you." I can still hear her voice.

Mom was one of my biggest supporters. In the years that followed my injury, I would call home to tell her about my life as a brain injury advocate on the road. "Mom, we're in Seattle," I'd share, my excitement palpable. She loved hearing about our many adventures. There is no better feeling than knowing that you've made your mom proud!

In the weeks between her funeral and upcoming burial, my PTSD has come back with a vengeance. It did the same thing after Mom's stroke last year.

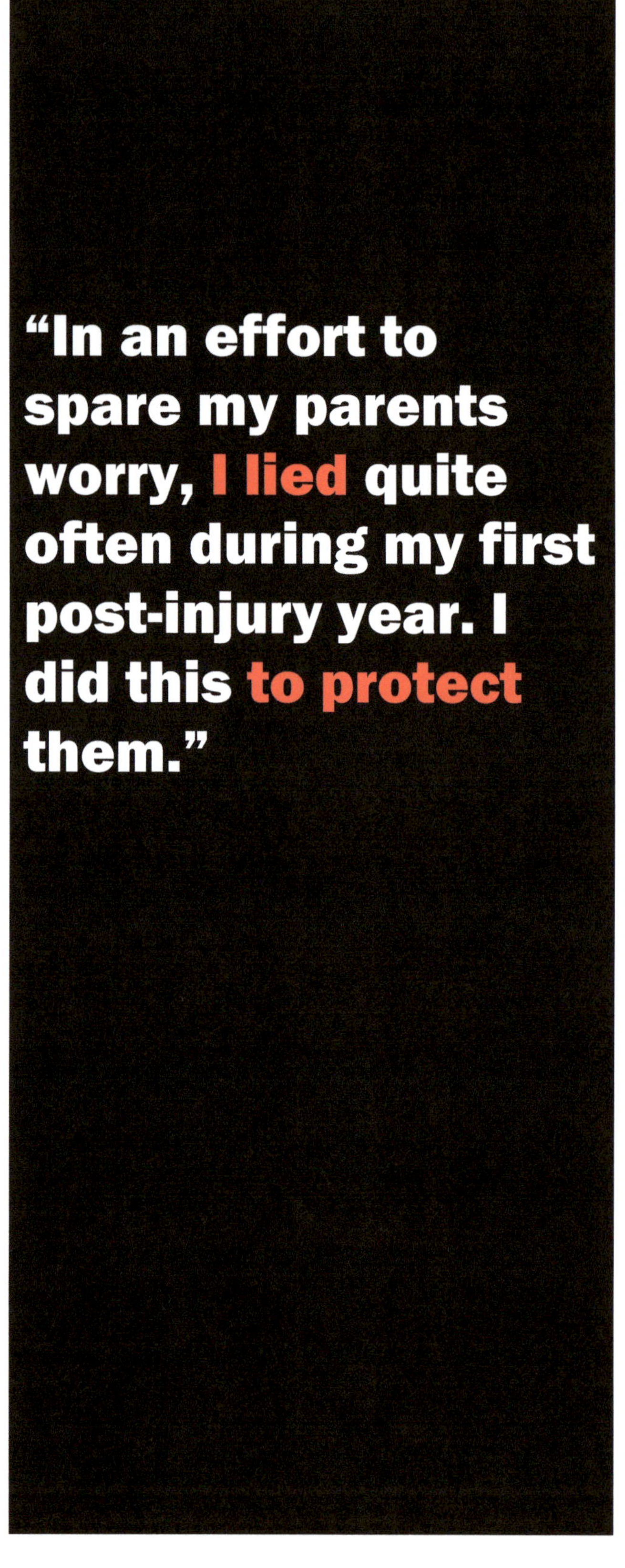

As my trauma doctor told me, "New trauma exacerbates old trauma." I fully expect this latest resurgence to pass as the weeks pass. I'm holding onto my seat on this roller coaster ride that so often accompanies life with both a TBI and PTSD.

There is still that utter disbelief that she's gone, a level of almost undefinable surrealism. I have a mom-shaped hole in my heart. My mom was 83 when she passed away as a direct result of a neurological condition. Not a day goes by that my eyes don't fill with tears.

We were at the rehab just a couple of short days before she died. Fate saw fit that we stayed for hours that day, much longer than our typical visits. Thank goodness for small miracles. We talked quietly in the common room and enjoyed the extra time just "being" in her company. I gave her an extra-long hug as we prepared to leave.

My last words to Mom, like they always were … "I love you, Mom."

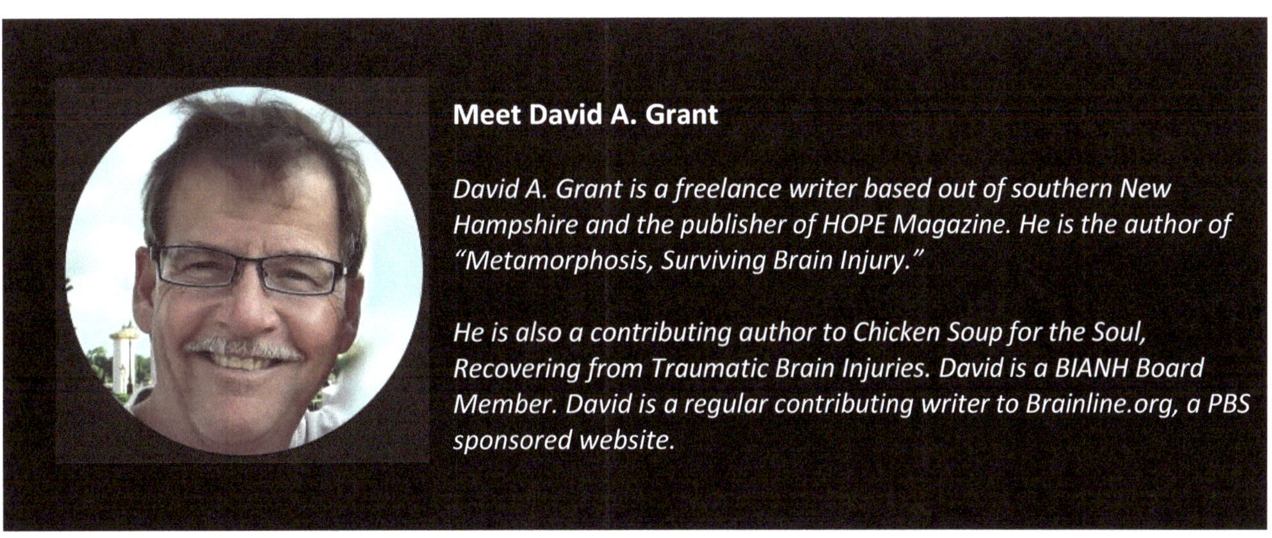

Meet David A. Grant

David A. Grant is a freelance writer based out of southern New Hampshire and the publisher of HOPE Magazine. He is the author of "Metamorphosis, Surviving Brain Injury."

He is also a contributing author to Chicken Soup for the Soul, Recovering from Traumatic Brain Injuries. David is a BIANH Board Member. David is a regular contributing writer to Brainline.org, a PBS sponsored website.

Living With Hope

By Patrick Brigham

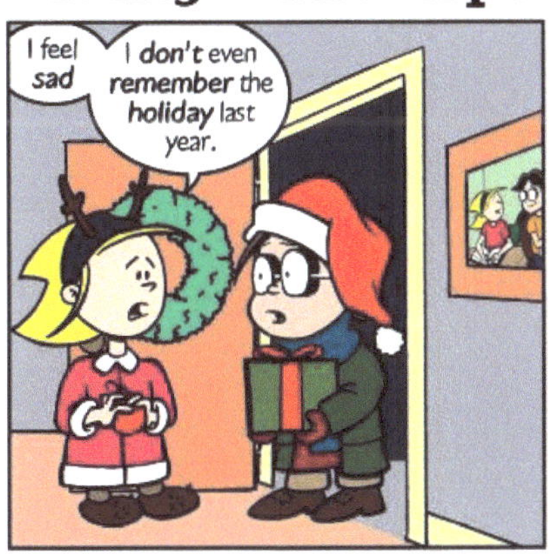

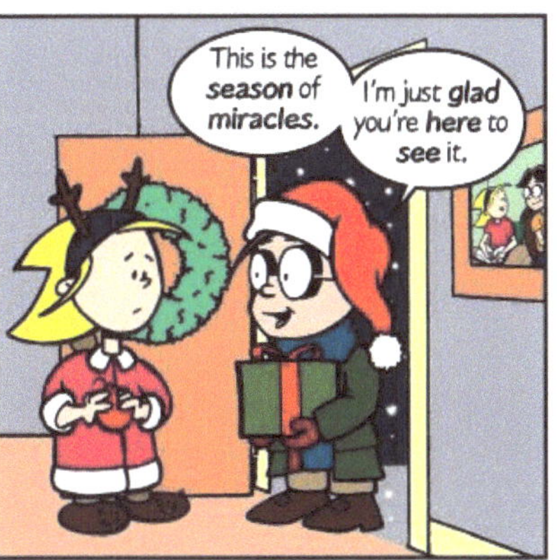

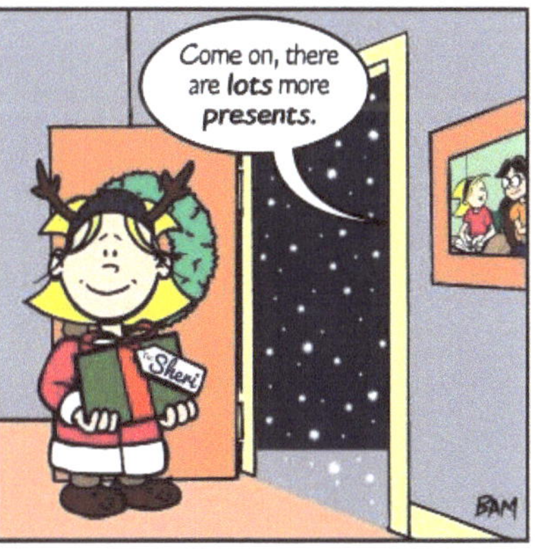

Front and Center

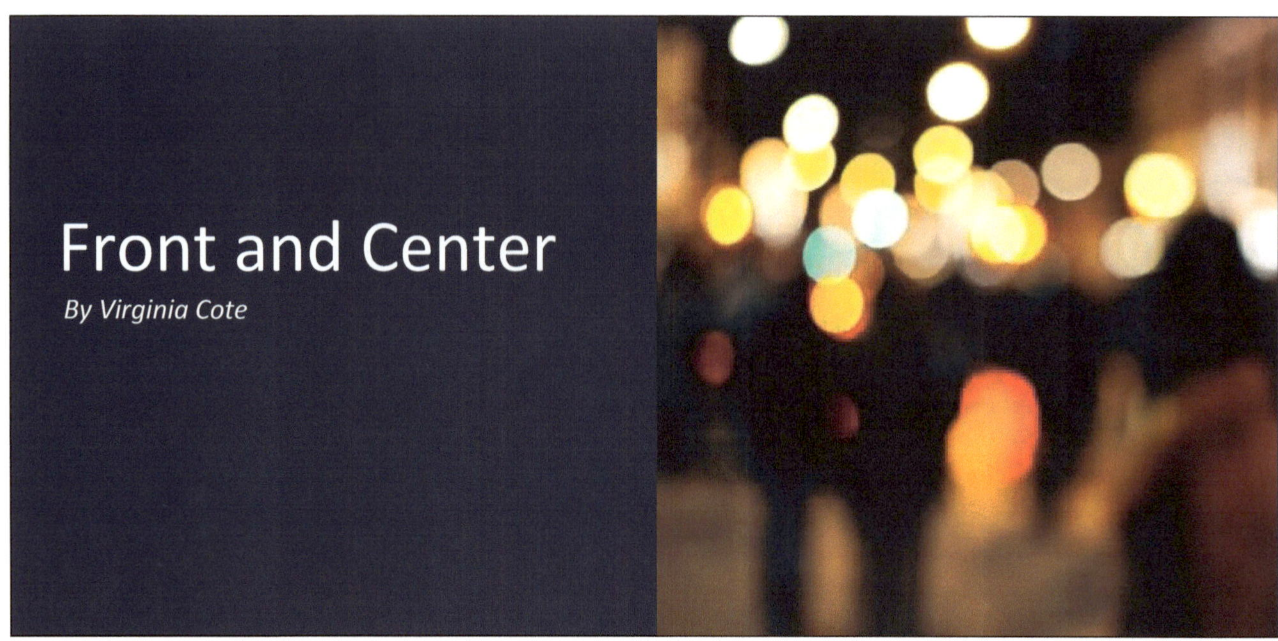

By Virginia Cote

"He looks normal." How many times have I heard that? I don't know what people expect to see when I say, "My son has a brain injury," and neither do they. It isn't anything to be embarrassed about. It isn't anything he wanted or asked for. It just happened. He was born with a defect in his head and at age forty-five the crimped blood vessels in his brain began to bleed and resulted in his brain damage. I have come to see that it is like his old life has ended and he has to begin a new life. That first year was a real battle. He wanted what he had lost but he could not capture it back. He fought to figure things out and to come to terms with his new self.

> *"I was aware that we were holding up a line of shoppers from entering but I needed to calm Rod. Not one person complained."*

Right from the start my son, Rod was right up front about his condition. Rod would go into a store looking for something and not be able to find the words when asking for help so he would say, "I have a brain injury. It is hard to find my words." He would continue to talk while hunting for the right words. Most times but not always, people would be very patient as they tried to help him to explain what he wanted. Both sides would smile when they accomplished the task.

Rod lived in Oregon when his bleed happened but soon moved back to New Hampshire with me. I am so thankful that I found Hope Magazine. This was really the only information I found on what Rod was going through and on what I could do to help him adjust and grow. Thank goodness for this publication.

Our first challenge and my first lesson were at Wal-Mart. We were headed in the door and I said we need to get this, this and this. Rod freaked out, I had overloaded him, and he wanted to go home. I stopped him right there in the doorway blocking it off completely. I said, "Rod stop, look at me, just look at me. We are only going to get this, this one item. Don't think about anything else. Can you do

that?" He agreed and we entered the store. I was aware that
we were holding up a line of shoppers from entering but I
needed to calm Rod. Not one person complained. They
quietly waited and gave us space. I wanted to hug every one
of them but needed to stay focused on Rod. I think by not
hiding the fact that he had a problem and by me calmly
helping Rod through it; that the line of shoppers was willing
to give up some of their time.

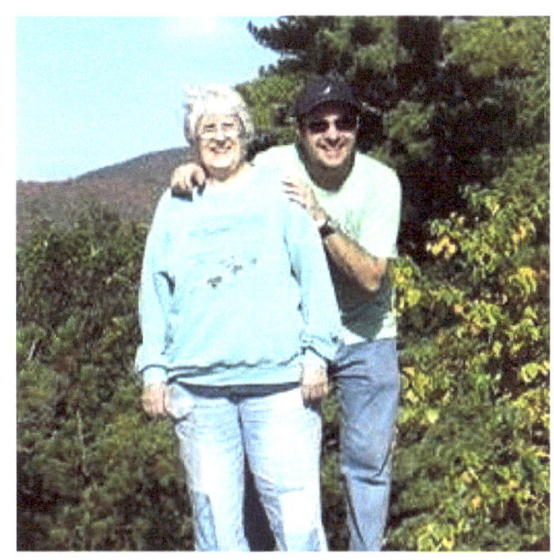

My next lesson was at a restaurant. Rod, my brother and I met
for dinner. The waitress came over asking if we were ready to
order. I didn't realize how bad Rod's reading, eyesight and
comprehension were at that point. The waitress began to rattle off the specials. Rod spoke up and
said, "I have a brain injury, can you go slow?" The waitress immediately talked right to Rod and
slowly explained everything to him. Whenever she returned to our table she would talk to Rod; then
to us. Rod figured out his brain injury couldn't be seen so he needed to let people know about it and
let them know how they could help but of course his thinking couldn't put those thoughts into words.
It was more instinct.

One of Rod's challenges was walking downtown along the busy road. It was very scary for him, but
he did not give up. Once downtown he visited the shops and got to know the owners. Always he
explained his injury and educated them. One stop was the community center. He went in often asking
if there were any programs for him. Finally, they said he could have coffee with the Senior Citizen
Group each morning. The seniors immediately took to him and admired his attitude. I tend to forget
and go too fast for Rod, but he patiently reminds me, "Mom you are overloading me." I try to break
things down for him. I am slowly learning instead of asking him to get something out of the car and
put it in the hall on the shelf for me to just ask if he can get something out of the car for me. Then I
wait for him to ask where I want it. I let him process the first request and then I let him ask when he
is ready for more directions.

Rod is not embarrassed about his injury; he puts it right out there before anyone can form wrong
ideas about what is going on with him. Rod does not accept he is unseen. He puts himself out there
front and center. He is educating the public. I know not everyone can do as Rod does but the more of
us that talk about it; the more the public will be comfortable around brain injuries. Most people just
don't know how to react or what they should do. The days of hushing it up and pretending it doesn't
exist are over.

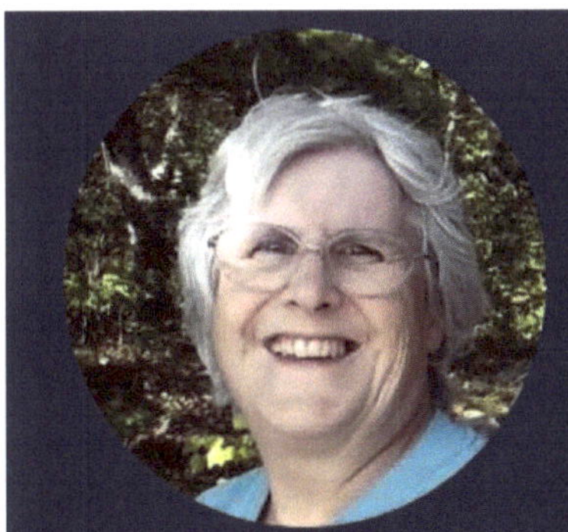

Meet Virginia Cote

Virginia Cote owns and operates a boarding and grooming kennel in New
Hampshire. When her son sustained his brain injury, she had no idea what
this would entail. She was in a fog for days and months. As she learned
more about brain injuries the fog slowly cleared and she found she could
indeed help her son.

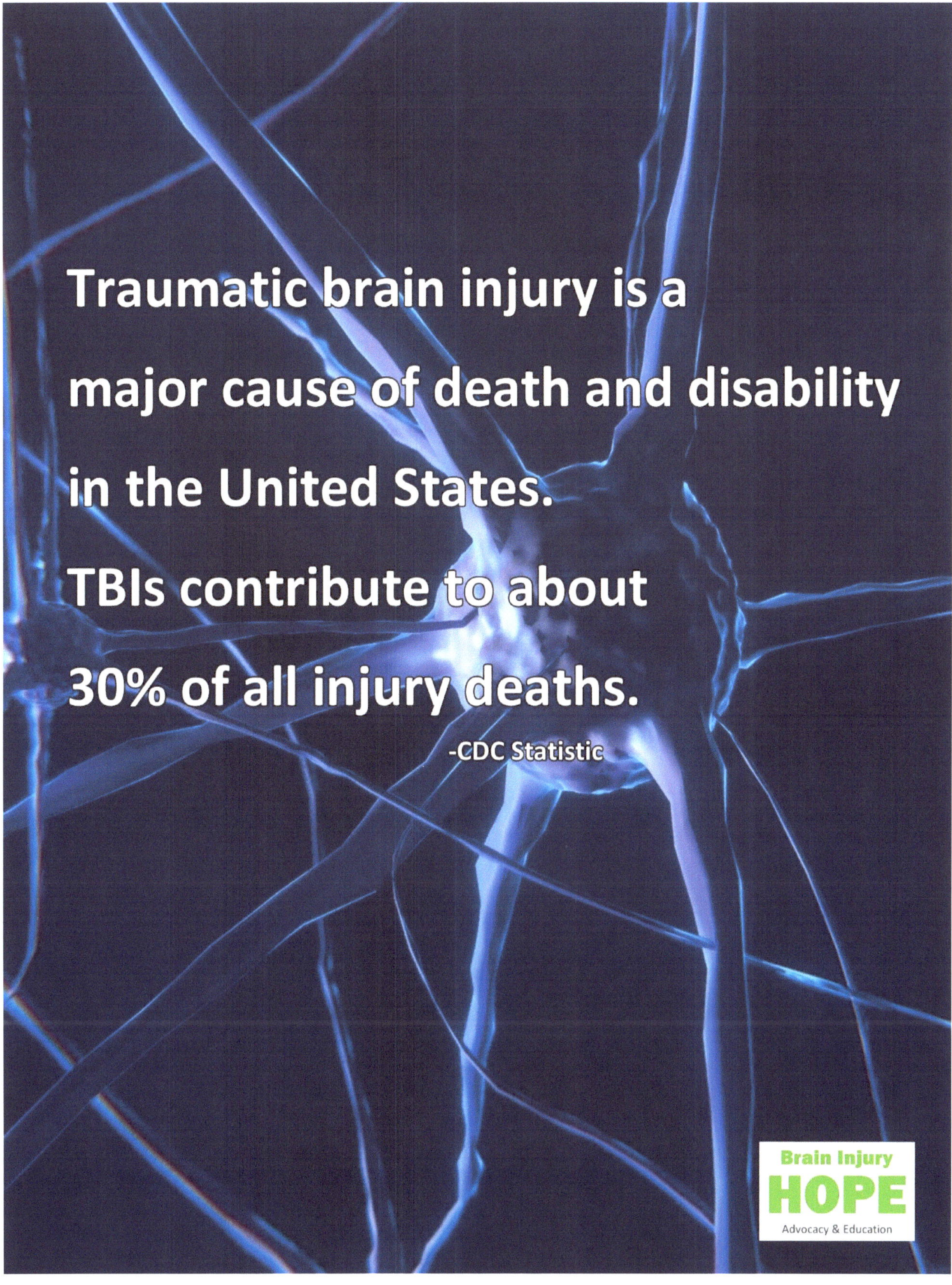

Traumatic brain injury is a major cause of death and disability in the United States. TBIs contribute to about 30% of all injury deaths.
-CDC Statistic
Brain Injury
HOPE
Advocacy & Education

What Are They Thinking?

By Jeff Sebell

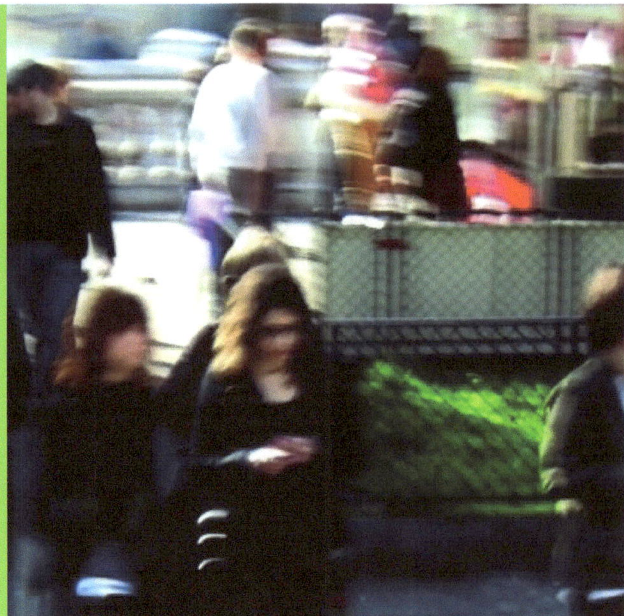

Sometimes people question what's wrong with us and say such blow-me-out-of-the-water unbelievable things that we are struck dumbfounded; unable to respond.

We are first made numb by the ignorance/unreality of what was just said. Add to that the fact that many of us have trouble processing information or shifting gears in conversations, and the result is we cannot think of, or articulate, a way to answer.

After a suitable amount of time has passed to figure out what actually happened, we might cry out passionately, "You don't understand!" and then get into some kind of argument. Sometimes, we might launch into an attempt to explain. This always a bad idea given the heat of the moment and our exasperation.

We take these things very seriously. When this happens, we feel as though our very essence is being attacked, and we feel a burning need to defend ourselves and clear our good name!

"People's reactions to the things we say and the things we sometimes do, their quick quips and offhanded statements, reinforce all the bad stuff we think about ourselves."

Only on those rare occasions when we are able to use all our power to restrain ourselves from impulsively answering, are we able to simply walk away, shaking our heads and muttering under our breath. We walk away, wondering how they could say something so ignorant, or stupid, or mean.

People's reactions to the things we say and the things we sometimes do, their quick quips and offhanded statements, reinforce all the bad stuff we think about ourselves. Rather than build us up when we really need a boost in confidence, other people often send us spiraling down into despair and depression.

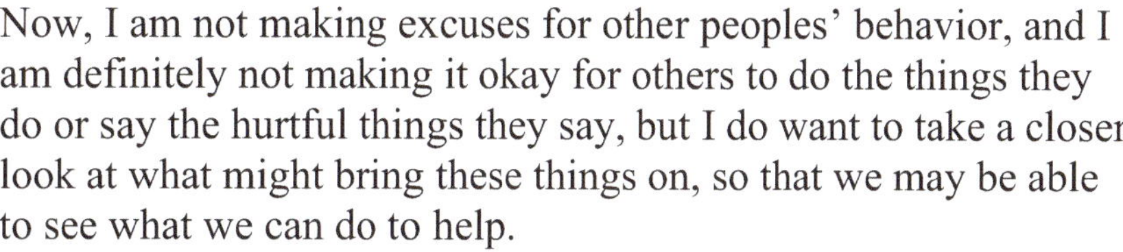

Now, I am not making excuses for other peoples' behavior, and I am definitely not making it okay for others to do the things they do or say the hurtful things they say, but I do want to take a closer look at what might bring these things on, so that we may be able to see what we can do to help.

We need to take a closer look at the dynamics here. The situation is this: it might help us to understand why others behave the way they do, by first examining what kind of impact we have on them.

Interpersonal communication is never simple, although we tend to see it as simple. In our minds, we have been knocked for a loop by a brain injury and, while not necessarily looking for sympathy, what we are asking for is some understanding and support. Something to make our lives easier.

"What could be simpler than that?" we ask.

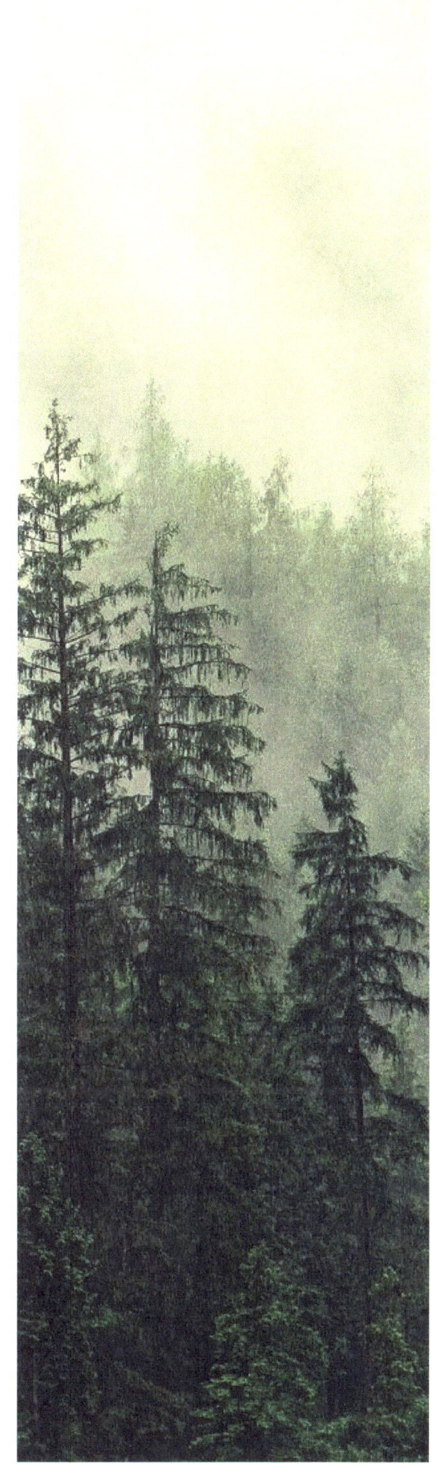

Let's look at the affect we have on others. Why don't we imagine you are walking down the sidewalk and a friend of yours comes up, approaching you from the other direction. What do you think is going through their mind when they see you?

Well, this person might be feeling uncomfortable, or have concerns or pity for this friend (you), who just doesn't seem right since his injury. Maybe he doesn't know how to be a friend in this situation and because of that, he feels like he is letting you down, so he feels bad and doesn't know what to say.

In the end he just really wants to help but is not sure how. After all, he really doesn't understand why things can't be the way they used to, and this makes him feel helpless.

He isn't really sure what to do, and truthfully, some things this person says to you might be an attempt to "jumpstart" you, sort of like giving you a little, well-meaning "kick in the pants". Just something to get you moving in the right direction. He may not mean to be hurtful, but it comes out sounding that way.

Beyond not knowing what to do, there is a question of expectations. You are expecting support from this friend or family member who doesn't know what to do. You expect your friend to be there to help out as you transition to normal life, but even you don't know what that means. There are expectations and confusions on both sides, and a once-clear friendship with boundaries and structure is now murky and cloudy.

In my own situation, after my neuropsych exam, I sat down with my parents and went over the report with them in detail to help them understand what was going on with me. When we want others to understand but don't give them the tools, we are setting ourselves up for failure. The only thing that is really clear is that we cannot be relying on others to set things right in our lives. This is not their fault. The responsibility for a relationship cannot be all on one side's shoulders.

As frustrating as it might be, it is your responsibility to teach. Collectively, it is our responsibility to instruct. Sometimes people question what's wrong with us and say such blow-me-out-of-the-water unbelievable things that we are struck dumbfounded; unable to respond.

We are first made numb by the ignorance and unreality of what was just said. Add to that the fact that many of us have trouble processing information or shifting gears in conversations, and the result is we cannot think of, or articulate, a way to answer.

After a suitable amount of time has passed to figure out what actually happened, we might cry out passionately, "You don't understand!" and then get into some kind of argument. Sometimes, we might launch into an attempt to explain. This is always a bad idea given the heat of the moment and our exasperation.

We take these things very seriously. When this happens, we feel as though our very essence is being attacked, and we feel a burning need to defend ourselves and clear our good name!

Only on those rare occasions when we are able to use all our power to restrain ourselves from impulsively answering, are we able to simply walk away, shaking our heads and muttering under our breath.

We walk away, wondering how they could say something so ignorant, or stupid, or mean.

People's reactions to the things we say and the things we sometimes do; their quick quips and offhanded statements, reinforce all the bad stuff we think about ourselves. Rather than build us up when we really need a boost in confidence, other people often send us spiraling down into despair and depression.

Now, I am not making excuses for other peoples' behavior, and I am definitely not making it okay for others to do the things they do or say the hurtful things they say, but I do want to take a closer look at what might bring these things on, so that we may be able to see what we can do to help.

We need to take a closer look at the dynamics here. The situation is this: it might help us to understand why others behave the way they do, by first examining what kind of impact we have on them.

Interpersonal communication is never simple, although we tend to see it as simple. In our minds, we have been knocked for a loop by a brain injury and, while not necessarily looking for sympathy, what we are asking for is some understanding and support. Something to make our lives easier.

"What could be simpler than that?" we ask.

Let's look at the affect we have on others. Why don't we imagine you are walking down the sidewalk and a friend of yours comes up, approaching you from the other direction. What do you think is going through their mind when they see you?

Well, this person might be feeling uncomfortable, or have concerns or pity for this friend (you), who just doesn't seem right since his injury. Maybe he doesn't know how to be a friend in this situation and because of that, he feels like he is letting you down, so he feels bad and doesn't know what to say.

In the end he just really wants to help but is not sure how. After all, he really doesn't understand why things can't be the way they used to, and this makes him feel helpless.

He isn't really sure what to do, and truthfully, some things this person says to you might be an attempt to "jumpstart" you, sort of like giving you a little, well-meaning "kick in the pants". Just something to get you moving in the right direction. He may not mean to be hurtful, but it comes out sounding that way.

Beyond not knowing what to do, there is a question of expectations. You are expecting support from this friend or family member who doesn't know what to do. You expect your friend to be there to help out as you transition to normal life, but even you don't know what that means. There are expectations and confusions on both sides, and a once-clear friendship with boundaries and structure is now murky and cloudy.

In my own situation, after my neuropsych exam, I sat down with my parents and went over the report with them in detail to help them understand what was going on with me. When we want others to understand but don't give them the tools, we are setting ourselves up for failure. The only thing that is really clear is that we cannot be relying on others to set things right in our lives. This is not their fault. The responsibility for a relationship cannot be all on one side's shoulders.

As frustrating as it might be, it is your responsibility to teach. Collectively, it is our responsibility to instruct.

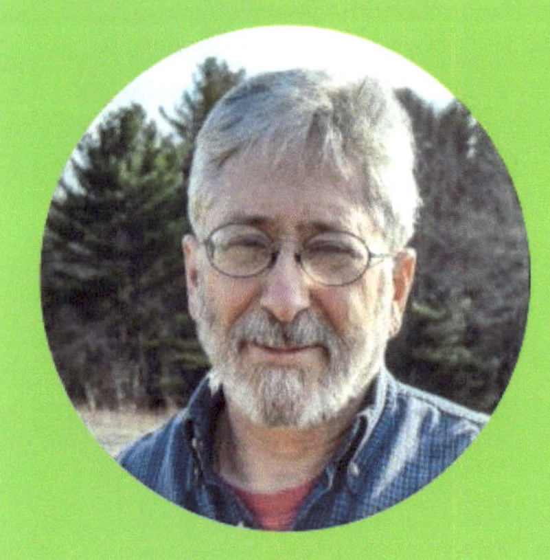

Meet Jeff Sebell

Jeff is a nationally published author, keynote speaker and blogger - writing about Traumatic Brain Injury and the impacts of his own TBI which he suffered in 1975 while attending Bowdoin College.

His book "Learning to Live with Yourself after Brain Injury," was released in August of 2014 by Lash Publishing.

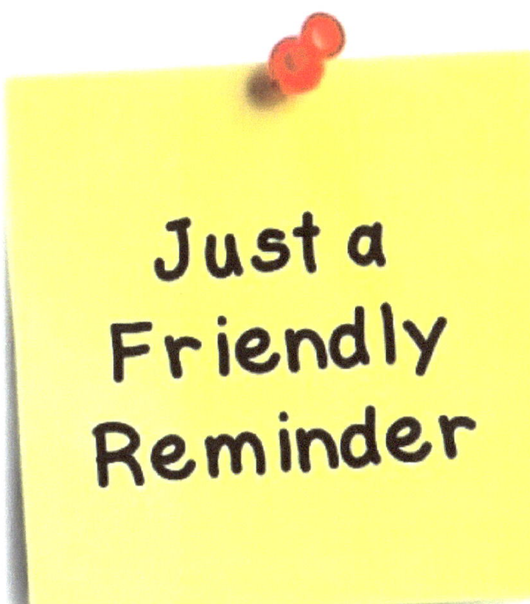

Starting in 2020 HOPE Magazine Will Be Published On a Quarterly Basis!

You can expect the same hope and inspiration you've come to love over the years in even larger volumes with more stories than ever!

Join our Facebook Family

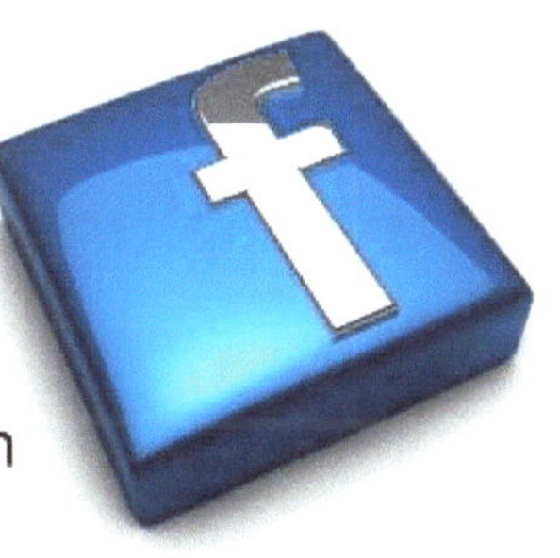

What do almost 30,000 people from 60 countries and five continents all have in common? They are all members of our vibrant Facebook family at /TBIHopeandInspiration

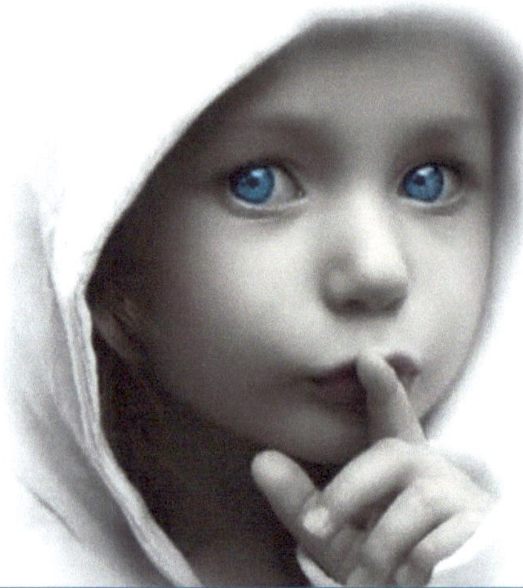

The Paradox of Silence

If I remain silent, my words will not betray me.

If I remain silent, my confusion remains within.

If I remain silent, I won't say something that I regret (again).

If I remain silent, no one can see that I am disabled.

If I remain silent, no one can hear my Soul cry.

If I remain silent, I can walk among the 'uninjured' without drawing attention.

If I remain silent, those who knew me 'before' will see no change.

If I remain silent, I will dwell alone in isolation.

If I remain silent, no one will ever know.

If I remain silent, those who can help me never hear my cries.

If I remain silent, I shut myself off from the love and help of others.

I am destined to never move forward...

If I Remain Silent

Your story has value. Kindly consider submitting your story for publication.

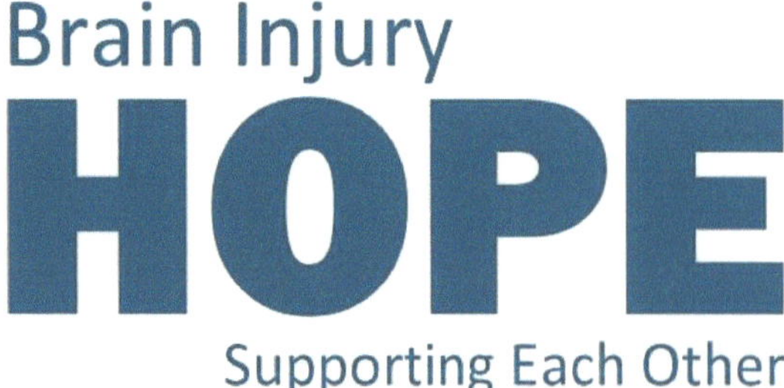

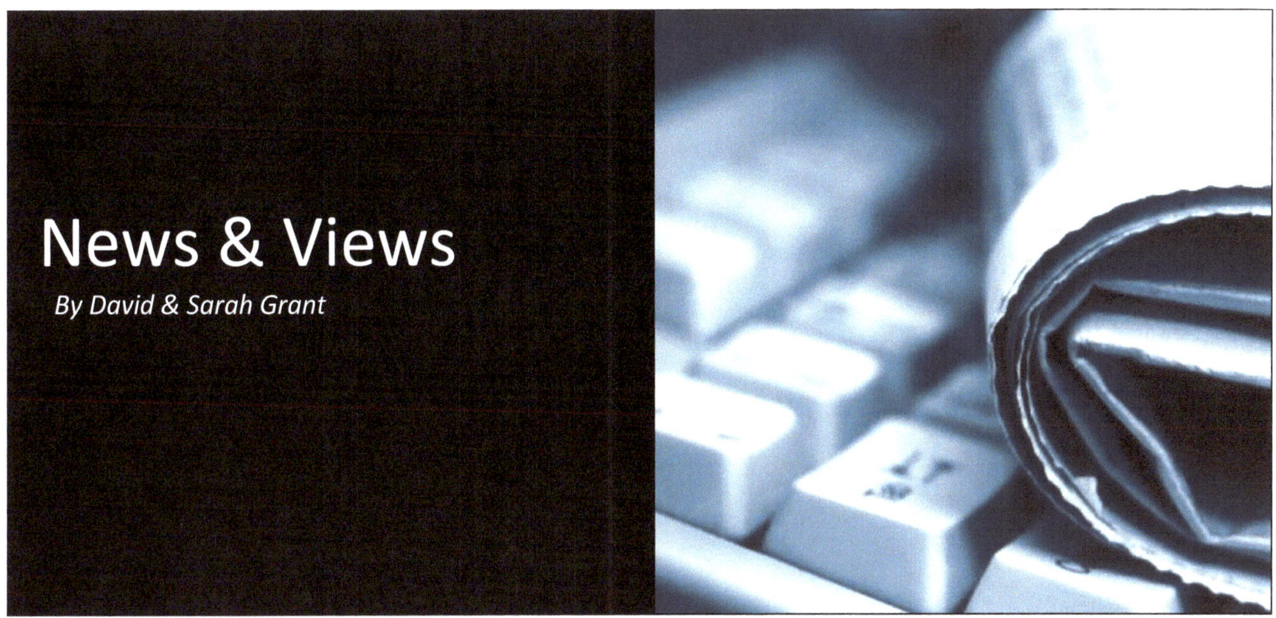

News & Views

By David & Sarah Grant

This past year has been one of both losses as well as surprising gains. Both Sarah and I lost our moms in 2019, Sarah's mom passing away unexpected in February, and my own mom passing away in September. Other family losses have made 2019 perhaps our most loss-filled year ever.

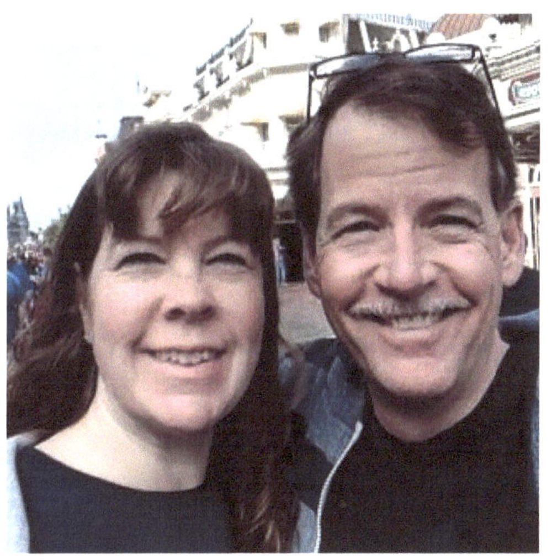

But there were also highlights that came unexpectedly, and in a few instances, quite surprisingly. A long-lost family member became part of our lives again, bringing with him a new and unexpected branch on our family tree. An upcoming wedding for one of our children will bring even more love into our sacred circle of life.

Brain injury did not stop our lives, nor did it slow down the inevitable circle of life that we are all part of.

Not as a survivor family, but rather of being part of the human family, it is critical that we be mindful of what we focus on. To dwell in all that has been lost bleeds the joy and hope out of today. Life passes all too quickly.

It is our hope that you are able to spend some time this holiday season with people who love you unconditionally, and who accept you as you are.

From our family to yours, Happy Holidays!

~ David & Sarah

www.ingramcontent.com/pod-product-compliance
Lightning Source LLC
Chambersburg PA
CBHW041136260726
48664CB00027B/1222